ADVANCE CARDIAC LIFE SUPPORT

Short, Sweet and to the Point

HELEN CARTER

BALBOA.PRESS

A DIVISION OF HAY HOUSE

Balboa Press books may be ordered through booksellers or by contacting:

Balboa Press
A Division of Hay House
1663 Liberty Drive
Bloomington, IN 47403
www.balboapress.com
1 (877) 407-4847

ISBN: 978-1-9822-4851-2 (sc)
ISBN: 978-1-9822-4852-9 (e)

Library of Congress Control Number: 2020911282

Print information available on the last page.

Balboa Press rev. date: 10/29/2020

Contents

A Special Thanks To:

Elizabeth Walker, Training Center Coordinator
(E & B Health and Safety LLC)
For helping me through a difficult transition from Arizona to Dunnellon.
Thank you not only for helping me expand my abilities in BLS, ACLS, and PALS,
but also for your encouragement to broaden my scope of practice into becoming a
Trauma Nursing Core Course and Emergency Nursing Pediatric Course Instructor.
Elizabeth is a unique individual who has touched the lives
of others in ways of which she is unaware.

Martha Mitchell, RN/BLS Instructor
Thank you
For taking me under your wing,
For always listening, and for your continuous encouragement:
"You Go Girl. You Got This."

Christian Diaz, Paramedic
CPR Program Administrator
CPR Training Shands, University of Florida
Thank you.
For being there:
Whenever, I've needed a sounding board or just someone to talk to.
You are always there to share our teaching and learning experience.
I truly appreciate you and thank you, for reading and helping me edit,
This Book!

Overview; the Science

High Quality Compressions, the Key to Success!

- BLS is the basic foundation to ACLS.
- Without good BLS your ACLS outcome will remain poor.
- Early CPR keeps oxygen-rich blood flowing and helps to delay brain damage and death.
- Immediately (within 10 seconds) start compressions push fast and push hard.
- At least 2 inches deep (AHA/ARC recommends the use of feedback devices no > 2.4.)
- Rate 100-120 / min (15-18 seconds to provide 30 compressions.)
- Allow for total recoil – Do not lean on the chest!
- Shock as soon as De-fib/AED is available, then every 2 minutes for VF or p VT.)
- Early defibrillation helps to restore an effective heart rhythm and significantly increase the patient's chance for survival.
- Minimize interruptions in compressions (no longer than 10 seconds off the chest.)
- Coronary Perfusion Pressure is the reflection of myocardial blood flow (difference in aorta and right atrial diastolic pressure.)
- Chest Compression Fraction (CCF)/CCR Chest Compression Rate is an indication of CPR quality.
- CCF/CCR is the percentage of time on the chest, doing compressions.
- Maintaining (CPP) > 20 mm Hg and a CCF /CCR > 60 (goal 80%) improves, pt. outcome.
- Pressures fall when compressions stop and time is needed to return to optimal pressures when, restarted.
- Integrate Post-Cardiac Arrest Care improves pt. outcomes.

Extracorporeal CPR

- Extracorporeal CPR refers to a cardiopulmonary bypass, which maintains organ perfusion while cardiac arrest causes are addressed.
- Is performed with an extracorporeal membrane oxygenation device. It includes a venous cannula, a pump, an oxygenator, and an arterial cannula
- Extracorporeal CPR is not recommended for routine use in cardiac arrest.
- Consider extracorporeal CPR when conventional CPR is failing and if providers are skilled and can implement it quickly.

Ventilations

- Avoid excessive ventilations, as it decreases cardiac output and cerebral perfusion.
- Avoid pneumothorax a complication, of B-M-V.

- Tidal volume 500-600 ml (some resources say 400-700 ml.)
- Just enough breath to see chest rise
- About ½ of the B-M-V

Early Recognition and Treatment

- Unable to maintain their own airway
- Respirator rate < 6 or > 30
- HR < 40 or > 140/min
- Systolic B/P < 90, MAP < 65
- Symptomatic hypertension
- Unexpected decrease LOC
- Unexpected agitation
- Seizures
- Significant decrease in Urine output
- Subjective concern about Pt.

Rapid Response Teams RRT/MET Medical Emergency Teams
Improve Patient Outcomes
By Identifying And Treating Early Clinic Deterioration

Access, Recognize and Care

- Is a concept that describes the ongoing process of gathering data about the patient's condition, using that data to identify a problem and then intervening to correct it ASAP
- It uses critical thinking, your past clinical experience and your general knowledge to correctly interpret the meaning of the data and gain an understanding of the patient's clinical situation and care needs
- Based on your understanding of the patient's condition, implement appropriate care.

Assess, Identify, Intervene, Reassess

Assessment Findings

- Taking a systematic approach to assessment allows you and the team to focus on identifying and addressing the most critical problems first.
- It also helps to ensure that important details about the patient's condition and underlying causes are not overlooked.

Systematic Approach includes rapid/primary and secondary assessments. The goal is early recognition and treatment.

Rapid Assessment is a quick visual survey to ensure safety, to form an initial impression about the patient's condition, to check for responsiveness, breathing and a pulse.

Initial Assessment helps you identify a situation as life/non-life threatening.

A - Appearance

- Responding/ unresponsive?
- Able to talk/cry

B - Breathing

- Are they breathing?
- Audible breath sounds
- Apneic

C - Color

- Do they have a pulse?
- Cyanotic/pale or mottled
- Any evidence of bleeding?

If Unconscious, call for help, not breathing, no pulse ....start compressions (BLS)

Conscious, in distress, call for help, when help arrives have them…VOMIT!!!

- V-Obtain Vital Signs,
- O-Check O_2 Sat,
- M-Get Them On The Monitor,
- I -Insert An IV/IO
- T-Treat Asap / Out Of Hospital T For Transfer

This systematic approach allows, the primary nurse to move quickly from the initial assessment to the primary assessment

Primary Assessment – (A B C D E), is a focused assessment of Airway, Breathing, Circulation, Disability and Exposure to identify potentially life -threatening conditions and address them immediately. This phrase allows for more advance treatment to stabilize the patient.

A-Airway

- Open the airway using either the head tilt chin lift or for suspected head/neck injury the jaw thrust
- Suction prn
- Insert OPA/NPA
- Consider an advance airway

B-Breathing

- Is it spontaneous?
- Rate-to fast/too slow?
- Depth and effort (regular/irregular)?
- Equal bilateral breath sounds/equal bilateral chest rise and fall
- O_2 sat maintain at > 94 % / capnography if available 35-45 %

C- Circulation

- Goal is to restore/maintain adequate perfusion.
- Pulse rate, quality and rhythm
- 12 lead EKG
- Cardiac monitor
- Systolic B/P > 90 fluids and/or pressers as indicated
- Cap refill
- Skin color, appearance and temperature

D – Disability

- LOC/A-V-P-U- Alert, Voice, Painful, Unresponsive
- Pupils – equal, round, reactive, light
- Glucose
- GCS/NIHSS

E- Exposure

- Remove clothing (rash, hives, S/S trauma, skin temperature)
- Signs of trauma or bleeding

Secondary Assessment – focus history and physical to establish a differential diagnosis and search/treatment causes

- S-Signs And Symptoms (Onset)
- A-Allergies
- M-Medication/OTC/Supplements
- P-Past Medical History
- L-Last Meal/Special Dietary Habits
- E-Events leading to illness or injury

H and T's

- Hypovolemia Tension Pneumothorax
- Hypoxia Tamponade (cardiac)
- Hyper/hypokalemia Thrombosis (Pulmonary/cardiac
- Hypothermia Toxins
- Hypoglycemia

Head To Toe Exam, Labs And Diagnostic Testing Are Included In the Secondary Assessment

- Anticipate what test will be needed
- Pain assessment and needs
- Pt/ Family support

High Quality BLS

Maintains Adequate Blood Supply To Brain and Vital Organs

- Scene Safety/Rapid Assessment a visual survey, Is it safe to approach the victim? What is your initial impression? Who's available? What do you need?
- Shout-Tap-Shout (Shout are you OK, Tap shoulders, Shout for help/911/AED)
- Assess, Recognize and Care is the systematic and continuous approach to life threatening emergencies.
- Use Systematic Assessment to determine unconsciousness/breathing
- Agonal Breaths are signs of a cardiac arrest
- Carotid pulse check at least 5-10 seconds
- Position the patient supine on a firm, flat surface and expose the patient's chest, then immediately begin chest compressions.
- Start compressions within 10 second.
- Push Fast, Push Hard!
- At least 2 inches deep …AHA/ARC recommends using a feedback device (no > 2.4.)
- Rate 100-120 minutes (15-18 seconds to perform 30 compressions.)
- Shoulders over the body, allow for total chest recoil, do not lean on the chest

- Minimize interruptions, no longer than 10 seconds off chest (including pauses for ventilations)
- Avoid excessive ventilations it decreases cardiac output and cerebral perfusion
- Compression to ventilation ratio 30:2
- Switch compressors every 5 cycles/about 2 minutes
- Use the AED/Monitor, as soon as it is available
- Turn it on first, then follow the prompts (continue compressions while charging)
- Most common mistake in CPR too many interruptions/too long off the chest
- Return to chest compressions ASAP after a shock!!!
- Maintaining (CPP) > 20 mm Hg and a CCF /CCR > 60 (goal 80%). Improves pt. outcome.
- Pressures fall when compressions stop and time is needed to return to optimal pressures

Recovery Position is used to help maintain a clear airway in an unresponsive patient who is uninjured and breathing normally

To Place An Adult In A Recovery Position:

- Kneel at the patient's side.
- Lift the patient's arm closest to you up next to their head.
- Place the patient's arm farthest from you next to their side.
- Grasp their leg closest to you, flex it at the hip and bend the knee toward their head.
- Place one of your hands on the patient's shoulder and your other hand on their hip farthest from you.
- Using a smooth motion, roll the patient toward you by pulling their shoulder and hip with your hands. Make sure the patient's head remains in contact with their extended arm.
- Stop all movement when the patient is on their side.
- Place their knee on top of the other knee so that both knees are in a bent position.
- Place the patient's free hand under their chin to help support their head and airway.

BLS for Children and Infants

Child Is 1- Puberty (Usually Around 12 Yrs. Of Age, Maybe Younger)

- Female-breast development
- Male chest or underarm hair
- Compressions on a child-about 2 inches (1/3 the depth of the chest)
- May use the heel of one hand for compressions
- S/S of poor perfusion with a HR< 60 begin compressions
- 30:2 for a single rescuer
- 15:2 for two rescuer

Infant under the Age of 1 Yrs. Old - we tap the bottom of their feet where as in adults/children you tapped their shoulders

- Pulse check in an infant is the branchial pulses vs the carotid in children/adult
- Compressions about 1.5 inches (1/3 the depth of the chest)
- S/S of poor perfusion with a HR < 60 begin compressions
- 30:2 for a single rescuer (two fingers)
- 15:2 for two rescuer (use thumb encircling technique) If unable to obtain proper depth, it is, acceptable to use the heel of one hand.

AED Use in Infant and Children

- Used only for a children under 8 years old
- Weights under 25 kg or 55 lbs.
- Pads placed front and back
- Never overlap pads
- Never cut pads
- Pads should never touch another
- If unavailable may use adult pads

Choking - Obtain Consent If Patient Is Alert)

Adult/Child (Responding)

- Abdominal thrust (while standing behind the person)

Infant (Responding)

- 5 Back slaps and 5 chest thrusts

Wheel Chair Bound

- For a person in a wheelchair start with chest thrust

Evidence suggests that it may take more than one technique to relieve an airway obstruction. If ineffective Back Blows and Chest Thrust for All Ages

Unresponsive choking (all ages)

- Call for help
- Begin compressions
- Prior to ventilation…look for obstructing objects

- See it….remove it
- No blind finger sweep

CPR Continues Until:

- ROSC
- Valid DNR
- Too exhausted to continue
- Scene becomes unsafe
- Other trained personnel arrive and relieve you

Measurements of High quality CPR
Team lead should assess for

- Minimize interruption no > than 10 seconds of the chest
- Compression are at the proper rate and depth
- Observe total chest recoil
- Observe ventilation are at the proper rate and volume
- Assess for compressor fatigue

Maternal Cardiac Arrest:

Follow ACLS treatments

- Same meds, defibrillation, early intubation
- CPR done with manual uterine displacement (pulled to the left side)
- 4 min until hysterotomy/ 5 min to delivery

A B C D E F G H - Differential Diagnosis for Maternity Arrests

- Anesthesia Complications
- Bleeding / DIC
- Cardiac disease/cardiovascular
- Drugs
- Embolism: Coronary / Pulmonary / Amniotic Fluid
- Fever
- General: PATCH 5 MD (or H's and T's
- Hypertension / preeclampsia / eclampsia

Amiodarone cannot be used on pts more than 20 weeks due to its, long half-life. Choose lidocaine instead!

Opioid Overdose

Respiratory Depression Is the Hallmark of Opioid Overdose Especially When Accompied by Unresponsiveness and Mitosis.

- Initiate high-quality compression first
- Ensure a patent airway / support ventilations
- O_2 Sat/Capnography
- IV/IO Access
- Give Naloxone; If effective repeated 4 minutes after the initial dose
- Although no evidence supports any benefit to naloxone administration during cardiac arrest, administration of naloxone during both respiratory and cardiac arrest is recommended when opioid overdose is suspected

Airway Management/Respiratory Arrest

A Patient Who Is Having Difficulty Breathing Requires Immediate Care.

- Respiratory distress can quickly progress to respiratory failure, respiratory arrest and cardiac arrest.
- In adults respiratory emergencies can have many underlying causes including disorders involving the respiratory, cardiovascular or nervous system
- Therefore, adequate respiration relies on the effective function of the respiratory system, cardiovascular system and the nervous system
- The respiratory system functions to provide the body's cells with oxygen and removes the byproduct of cellular metabolism, carbon dioxide (Oxygenation and ventilation)
- The diaphragm is the primary muscle responsible for ventilation. When ventilation demands increase, the body recruits accessory muscles for assistance.
- Expiration is a passive action that occurs when the diaphragm and external intercostal muscle relax
- Problems with ventilation occur in the presence of conditions that affect the body's ability to move air in and out of the lungs. (ex COPD, overdose)
- Respiratory distress represents the earliest stage on the continuum. A patient in respiratory distress is using compensatory mechanisms to maintain adequate oxygenation and ventilation
- If the patient's respiratory distress is not relieved, these compensatory mechanisms will soon become inadequate, at which point the patient may develop respiratory failure.
- Respiratory arrest is complete cessation of the breathing effort. The body can tolerate respiratory arrest for only a very short time before the heart stops functioning as well, leading to cardiac arrest

• Distress	• Failure	• Arrest
• Dyspnea • Inability to speak without pausing between words • Changes in breathing rate and depth use of assessor muscles • Bradycardia/tachycardia abnormal breath sounds (wheezing, crackles, rhonchi) • Diaphoretic • Petco > 45 % • Change in mental status	• PETCO greater than 50 mm hg • Decreased or irregular Respirtory rate • Change of level of conscious • SaO2 <90% • Cyanosis	• Loss of consciousness • No breath sounds • Lack of chest movement • Cyanosis/pallor • Bradycardia

Airway Management Is a Fundamental Lifesaving Skill

- Open the airway
- Jaw thrust for suspected head/neck injury
- Head tilt /chin lift with no injury
- OPA, unconscious pts or NPA, Semi-conscious, conscious or unconscious pts. Should be used to prevent the tongue from obstructing the airway.

Recue Breathing Is Breaths without Compressions

- 1 breath over about 1 second-look for chest rise and fall
- 1 breath q 6 seconds/10 BPM…Adults
- 1 breath q 2-3 second/20-30 BPM….Children and infants
- Avoid excessive ventilation – Gastric distention/potential vomiting and aspiration Increases intrathoracic pressure, Decreases venous return and cardiac output which decreases cerebral perfusion
- Tidal volume 500-600 ml (some resources say 400-700 ml)
- Just enough to see chest rise (squeeze bag about half way)

Advance Airway

Endotracheal Tube

- Offers complete protection of the airway from aspiration
- Facilitates tracheal suctioning

- Provides an alternate administration route for some medications
- Best choice when the need for long-term assisted ventilation is anticipated
- Cricoid Pressure- not routinely recommend (may be use if high risk of aspiration)

Confirmation of ET Tube

- Auscultation
- Chest rise and fall
- Colorimetric capnography (color change CO_2 detector)
- Continues waveform capnography
- ABGS/Chest X-Ra

CPR Cycle After Intubation 1 Breath Q 6 Seconds /10 BPM without Pausing Compressions

Laryngeal Mask Airway

- The laryngeal mask airway consists of an airway tube and a mask with an inflatable cuff at the distal end.
- The mask is advanced along the contour of the pharynx with the aperture of the mask facing the tongue until resistance is met.
- Properly positioned, the mask opening overlies the glottis, while the bottom rim wedges up against the upper esophageal sphincter, creating a seal.
- Once the cuff of the mask is inflated, the glottis is isolated, permitting air from the tube to enter the trachea.

ET Suctioning

- Hyper-oxygenate prior to suctioning
- Suction < 10 seconds
- Suction during withdrawal

When an advanced airway is in use, confirm its correct placement initially, whenever the patient is moved and on an ongoing basis.

Correct placement of an advanced airway is verified using both physical assessment (observing for bilateral chest rise and auscultating over the lungs and epigastrium) and a confirmation tool (such as capnography).

Fogging in the tube and ease of ventilation are not reliable methods of confirming correct advanced airway placement.

- **PETCO2**
- **Best indicator of CPR efficiency & coronary perfusion**
- **During CPR ≥10 goal 15-20**
- **Best indicator of ETT placement and monitoring**

Capnography vs. Oximetry

- Pulse oximetry measures oxygenation
- Capnography measures ventilation and provides a graphical waveform available for interpretation
- Capnography: the standard for monitoring intubated and non-intubated patients in a variety of settings.
- Capnography can be used in procedural sedation, CPR, ET Tube insertions & to check effectiveness of ventilator adjustment
- Capnography sensors can be placed at the airway exit – the nose, mouth or ET tube hub to measure ventilation.
- Capnography provides visual evidence of a patent airway within 15 seconds

Capnography

In The Intubated Patient, Can Be Used For:

- Verification of ET tube placement
- Continuous monitoring of ET tube position

In Cardiac Arrest Patient, Can Be Used For:

- To check effectiveness of cardiac compressions, it should read > 10 with the goal >15-20 mm Hg.
- First indicator of the return of spontaneous circulation even before the pulse or blood pressure change
- Normal capnography in ROSC is 35-45 mmHg

PETCO – Partial Pressure of Carbon Dioxide at the End of Expiration.

- Lungs transport O_2 to the cells where it is metabolized, CO_2 is transported via the blood to the lungs to be exhaled
- The amount of CO_2 in the exhaled gases is determined by alveolar ventilation, perfusion status and metabolic rate.

- It is the number value of the high point of the waveform, at the end of expiration.
- End-Tidal Carbon Dioxide values in the range of 35 to 45 mm/Hg confirm adequacy of ventilation.

Five Steps to Interpret a Waveform

- Is there a waveform?
  - Even an abnormal waveform shows that carbon dioxide is present

- Is the respiratory baseline flat and consistent from breath to breath?
  - A respiratory baseline that slopes upward and increases with each breath suggest that the patient is rebreathing carbon

- Look at the respiratory upstroke is the upstroke steep, sloping or prolonged?
  - A prolonged respiratory upstroke that is not vertical represents uneven alveolar emptying as a result of bronchospasm that obstructs the lower airway upon exhalation such as that seen in an asthma attack or COPD exacerbation

- Look at the expiratory plateau is the plateau flat, or completely absent?
  - A flat plateau indicates complete exhalation and emptying of carbon dioxide from the alveoli. This means that the PETCO reading is accurate and at peak levels (CO2 has been completely purged from the airway
  - Loss of the plateau is produced by uneven alveolar emptying secondary to severe bronchospasm that leads to air trapping
  - An absent plateau suggests dynamic hyperflexion also called auto positive end expiratory pressure (auto peep)

- Read the Petco value.
  - A measurement > 45 mm hg suggest hypercapnia which may be caused by respiratory failure
  - A measurement < 35 mm hg suggest hypocapnia which may be caused by hyperventilation or hypo perfusion

Normal Capnogram

- Consist of a flat baseline, a steep upstroke and down stroke, a flat plateau and Petco value between 35-45 mm hg a Sloped upstroke indicates pathology
- Knowledge of waveform characteristics enable provider to assess ventilation status.

A normal wave form has four phrases and a square shape

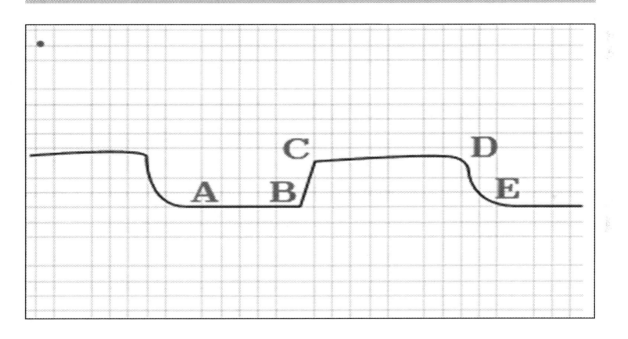

Hyperventilation

Normal   PETCO 45

RR ↑ PETCO ↓

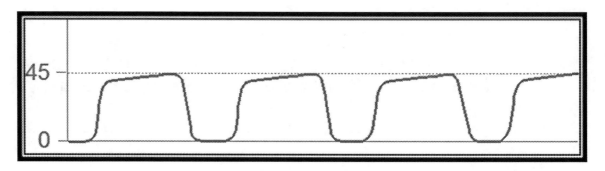

Hyperventilation

Hyperventilation   PETCO 30

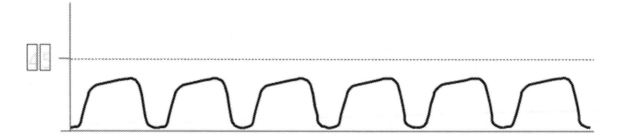

Hypoventilation

Normal   PETCO 45

RR ↓ PETCO ↑

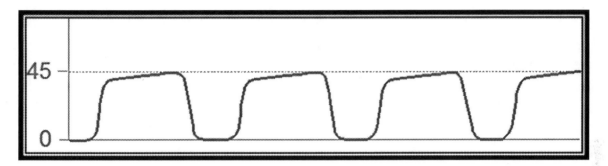

Hypoventilation   PETCO 60

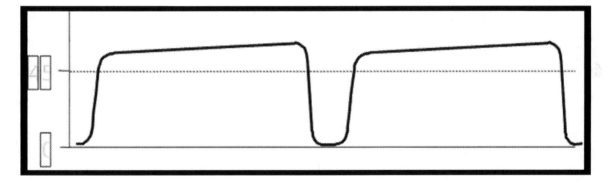

A SaO$_2$ level of less than 90% (PaO$_2$ of less than 50 mmHg) accompanied by PETCO$_2$ values greater than 50 mmHg is indicative of respiratory failure.

Which Segment On A Capnography Waveform Reflects The Beginning Of Exhalation?

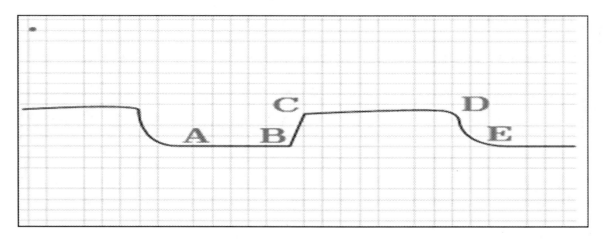

The A–B segment is the respiratory baseline, which represents the beginning of exhalation.

At Which Point On the Capnography Waveform Would the Patient's End-Tidal Carbon Dioxide (PETCO) Level Be Measured?

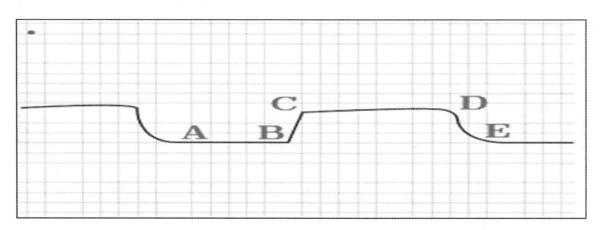

The PETCO value is measured at the end of exhalation
(point D), which represents the peak level.

Team Dynamics Elements of Team Dynamics and Communication

Communication It the Basic Foundation of Good Teamwork Team Dynamics Are Critical In a Code!!!!

- Sender/ team lead –speaks respectfully in a calm voice sending a clear message
- The receiver/team member hears and confirms the message was understood by providing feedback to the sender therefore closing the loop in the communication

Roles

- Clear roles and responsibilities
- Designated Team leader
- Know limitations
- Constructive intervention

What to Communicate

- Knowledge sharing
- Summarizing and reevaluation

How to Communicate

- Closed-loop communication
- Clear messages
- Mutual respect

Debriefing

During and After Resuscitation Attempts

- Work together as a team
- Debriefing during and after code
- Improves team performance
- Improves patient outcome after arrest
- Ex. statement during debriefing indicating that the team performed high quality CPR might be:

We delivered 1 ventilation every 6 seconds and chest compressions at a rate of 100 to 120 compressions per minute. With no interruptions in compressions for ventilations

Effective High-Performance Teams

- Debrief their performance after each resuscitation event.

The Purpose of Debriefing

- Is to review the decisions that were made and the actions that were taken to identify opportunities for improvement at system, team and individual levels.

Management of Arrhythmias

- Although not every cardiac arrhythmia is dangerous, many can be serious, and some require immediate treatment to prevent sudden death.

Primary Arrhythmias

- Occur with anatomically normal hearts and reflect an intrinsic abnormality of electrical cardiac conduction.

Secondary Arrhythmias

- Occur because of diseases affecting the heart or causing metabolic abnormalities, or due to drug effects.

Arrhythmias Can Be Classified

- Based on heart rate: too slow (Brady arrhythmias) or too fast (tachyarrhythmias).
- Arrhythmias can be further characterized by whether perfusion is adversely affected (unstable) or not (stable).
- Some arrhythmias are well tolerated and self-limiting, whereas others may cause decreased cardiac output with associated symptoms
- Prompt assessment, recognition and care of a patient with a cardiac arrhythmia may prevent deterioration to hemodynamic instability, which if untreated can result in shock, heart failure or cardiac arrest.

Algorithm's : Stable vs Unstable

- B/P too high/low
- Change in mental status
- Chest pain
- Acute heart failure

- Heart rate too fast/slow
- S/S shock

Assess Your Patient….A Talking Patient, Is Not Always STABLE…

15 Lead/12 Lead vs 5/ 3 Lead EKG

3 Lead EKG

- is usually for transport,
- it monitors two different areas of the heart one lateral and one inferior
- Non diagnostic as it does not provide a clear view of the entire heart

5 Lead EKG

- Is preferred in ICU as in addition to the inferior and lateral view it also gives you and anterior view
- A 5 lead provides a lot of information
- However if something concerned is noted a 12 lead should be done to provide even more information

12 Lead EKG

- Gives a detailed look at the hearts three areas

The 12 Lead EKG Consist Of:

- Three bipolar limb leads I, II, III
- The unipolar limb leads AVR, AVL,and AVF
- Six unipolar chest leads, also called precordial or V leads

15-Lead

- Diagnosis and Treatment of Right Ventricle and
- Left Ventricle Posterior and Lateral Wall

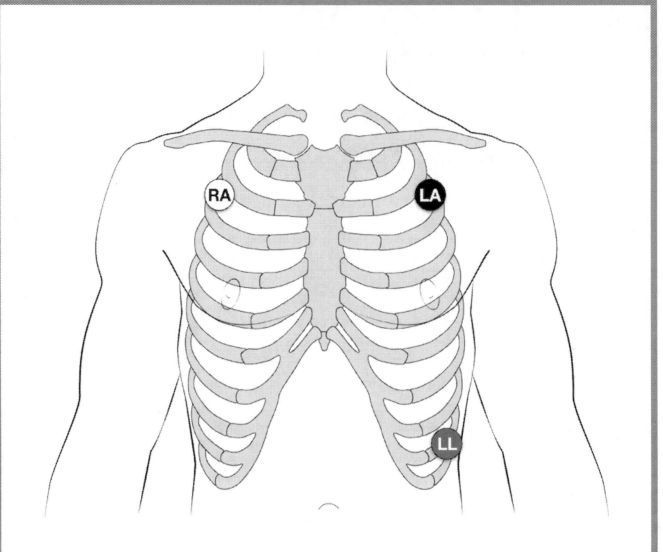

3 Lead EKG Placement

- White on right just below the clavicle (midway)
- black on left just below the clavicle
- Red is on the left of the lower edge of the rib cage

White on the Right, Smoke over Fire

Anatomical Location of Each Lead: Using a Five-Electrode System

- White is on the right side, just below the clavicle (midway)
- Black is on the left side just below the clavicle
- Brown is in the 4th intercostal space, just to the right of the sternum
- Green is on the right on the lower edge of the rib cage/ On the lower right abdomen
- Red is on the left of the lower edge of the rib cage

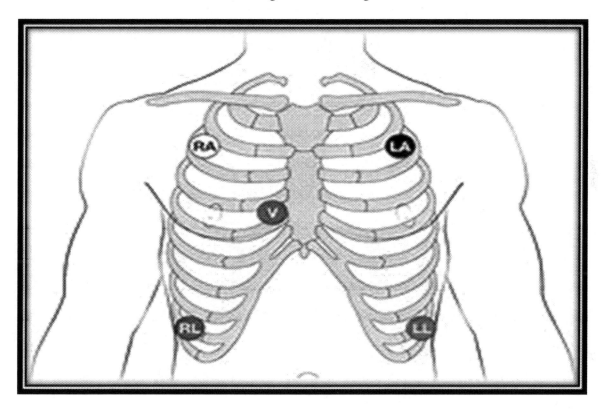

Snow over Grass, Smoke over Fire

12 Lead EKG (Lead Placement)

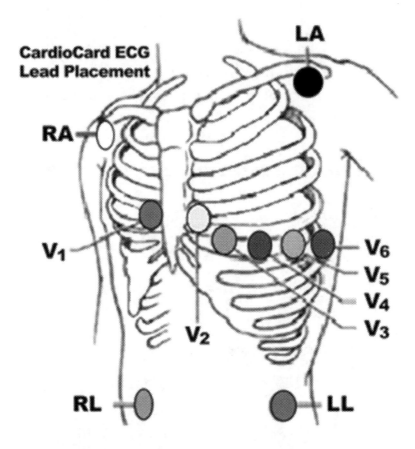

V1 - Fourth intercostal space on the right sternum

V2 - Fourth intercostal space at the left sternum

V3 - Midway between placement of V2 and V4 Fifth intercostal space at the midclavicular line

V5 - Anterior axillary line on the same horizontal level as V4

V6 - Mid-axillary line on the same horizontal level as V4

RA Right Arm - Anywhere between the right shoulder and right elbow

RL Right Leg - Anywhere below the right torso and above the right ankle

LA Left Arm - Anywhere between the left shoulder and the left elbow

LL Left Leg- Anywhere below the left torso and above the left ankle

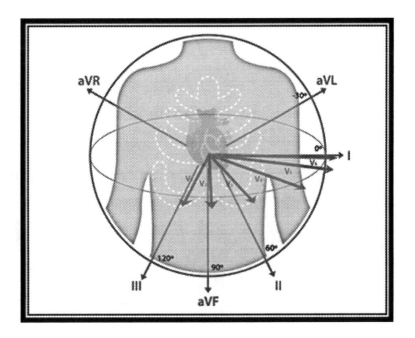

A Lead Is:

- A glimpse of the electrical activity of the heart from a particular angle.
- Put simply, a lead is like a perspective.

In 12-lead EKG

- There are 10 electrodes providing 12 perspectives of the heart's activity using different angles through two electrical planes.
- The vertical and horizontal planes.

Vertical plane (Frontal Leads)

- By using 4 limb electrodes, you get 6 frontal leads that provide information about the heart's vertical plane:

  - Lead I
  - Lead II
  - Lead III
  - Augmented Vector Right (aVR)
  - Augmented Vector Left (aVL)
  - Augmented vector foot (aVF)

- Leads I, II, and III require a negative and positive electrode (bipolarity) for monitoring. On the other hand, the augmented leads-aVR, aVL, and aVF-are unipolar and requires only a positive electrode for monitoring.

15 Lead EKG Placement

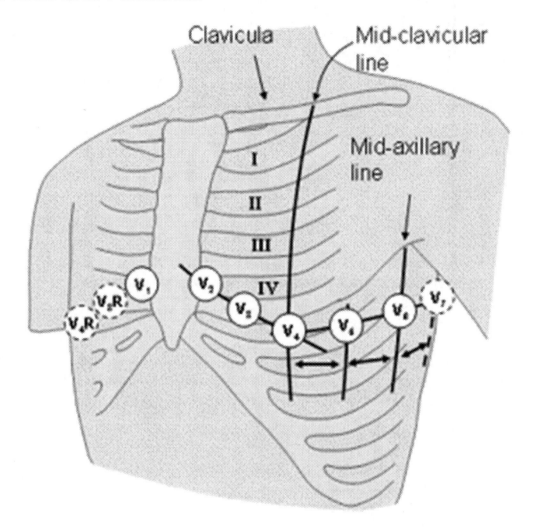

The EKG is a real time recording of the hearts electrical activity, as impulses travel through the conduction system causing depolarization and then repolarization of the hearts cells

The Cardiac Conduction System is a group of specialized myocardial cells that generate and transmit the electrical signals that cause the heart muscle to contract. A well-functioning conduction system is essential for ensuring the rhythmic, coordinated contraction of the heart that is necessary to maintain cardiac output

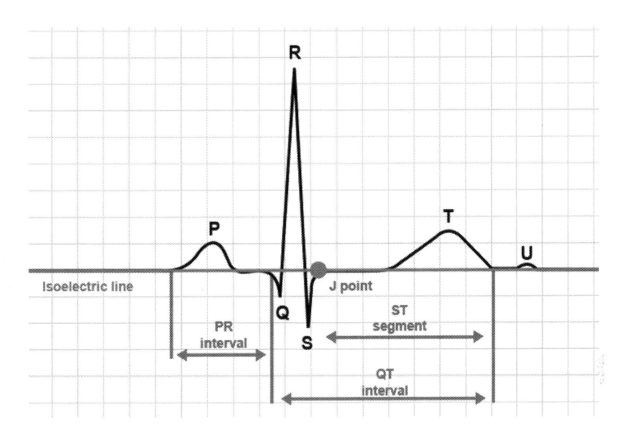

P Wave

- Represents atrial depolarization
- Produced by the SA node
- Normally upright
- Usually no more than 3 mm in height

PR Interval

- Measured from the start of the p wave to the beginning of the QRS.
- Normal duration 120-200 milliseconds **(.12-.20)**
- Represents the time of atrial depolarization to the beginning of QRS. depolarization

QRS. Complex

- Represents depolarization of the ventricular myocardial cells
- QRS. complex is less than 120 milliseconds **(.12)**
- Measured from the beginning of the QRS. to the end of the T-wave (time the ventricular depolarization to the end of repolarization
- QRS. is made up of
    - Q wave – 1st negative deflection from baseline

- R wave positive deflection from baseline
- S wave- negative deflection following the r wave

R prime is the secondary positive wave that may represent abnormal

Isoelectric Line —flat line of the EKG tracing represents no electrical activity, and referred to as the baseline

T Wave

- Represent ventricular repolarization as the ventricles return to a state of relation
- T-wave is normally upright but may vary if myocardial injury or ischemia is present
- Typically round and systematical

ST Segment

- Represents early ventricular repolarization
- Extends from the end of the QRS. to the beginning of the T-wave
- Normally even with the isoelectric line
- Deviation above or below the line indicate ; injury (elevation > 1 mm or Depression >1 mm ischemia in two or more reciprocal leads

QT Interval (Total Ventricular Activity)

- Represents the refractory period of the ventricles, as they depolarize and repolarize
- Begins at the 1st wave in the QRS. and ends when the T wave returns to baseline
- QT Interval is (0.36-0.40)seconds and directly relates to heart rate

J Point

- Point where the QRS. ends the ST segment begins
- J point elevation can be seen in early repolarization
- At times J point elevation can be ischemic, however this is somewhat rar

To Interrupt an EKG, Look At the Rhythm

- What is the rate, is it regular/irregular?
- Look at the P wave- is it present, upright (lead 2) all look the same. Do you only have one p for each QRS?
- Look at the QRS. - is it narrow or wide, same morphology?
- Look at T wave —all look alike (less than 5 mm in height)?

- Look at the PR- consistent/varies? Less than .20?
- Look at the QT interval, varies with heart rate- in general. > .46 is considered prolonged and never should be > 500 in pts on medication that can prolong the QT interval
- Prolonged QT Interval is associated with increased risk of torades.
- Look at the ST segment elevated/depressed

The Cardiac Conduction System Consists Of:

- Sinoatrial (SA) node,
- Atrioventricular (AV) node,
- Bundle of His, the left and right bundle branches
- Purkinje fiber

SA Node Also Called the Pacemaker of the Heart

- Located in wall of the right atrium
- These cells can spontaneously produce an electrical impulse
- The nerve impulses travel throughout the heart wall causing both of the atria to contract emptying blood into the ventricles before ventricular contraction
- SA node is Regulated by the Anatomic nerve system of the peripheral nervous system
- Parasympathetic and sympathetic autonomic nerve system send impulses to the SA node to either speed up SNS or to slow down PSNS the heart rate according to need
- Ex HR increases during exercise to keep up with increase O2 demand and returns to normal when exercising stops

AV node Lies on the right side of the partition that divides the atria near the bottom of the right atrium

- Acts to delay the impulses sent form them SA node for about a 10th of a seconds to ensure the atria has enough time to fully empty into the ventricles before ventricle systole
- The AV node then sends the impulses down the AV bundle of his to the ventricles
- AV node ensures the impulses do not move to rapidly which could cause A-fib

AV Bundle of His is a bundle of cardiac muscle fibers located within the septum of the heart, each bundle branch continues down the center of the heart and carries impulses to the right and left ventricle

- If there is a blocked near the hearts ventricles, the electric impulse may travel slightly longer to reach its endpoint. Making it harder to pump blood throughout the body.

- Right Bundle Branch Block (RBBB) is a blockages of the impulse at the right ventricle where as a blockage at the left ventricle is a LBBB

  - The Left branches into an anterior and posterior fascicles given rise to the Purkinje fibers
  - Bundle of his Transmits impulses from the AV node to the Purkinje

Purkinje Fibers specialized Purkinje fibers are a vital component in the functioning of the heart, and are thus, vital for our survival.

- They are found just beneath the endocardium (inner wall) of the ventricular extend from the AV bundle of his to the left and right ventricle
- They rapidly relay impulses to the myocardium (middle Layer) of the ventricles causing both ventricles to contract
- The myocardium is thickest in the ventricles which allows them to generate enough power to pump blood to the rest of the body
- The right ventricle forces blood along the pulmonary circuit to the lungs
- The left ventricle forced blood along the systemic circuit to the rest of the body
- Purkinje fibers have been implicated in both the maintainace and the initiation of tachyarrhythmia's
- The Purkinje network plays a pivotal role in both the imitation and perpetuation of VF

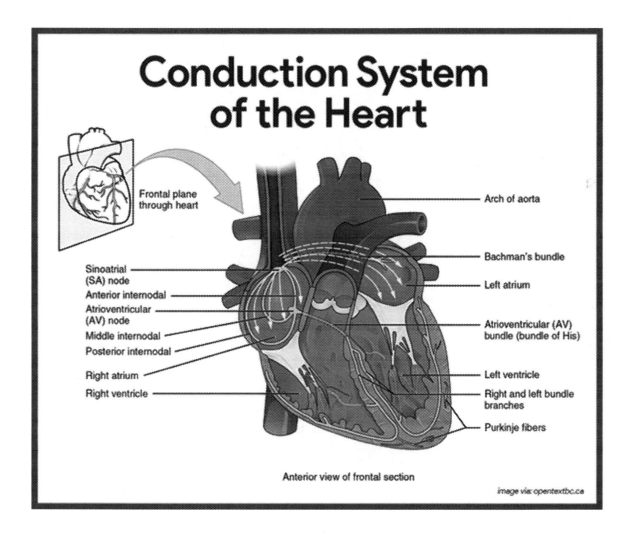

Conduction System of the Heart

Frontal plane through heart

Sinoatrial (SA) node

Anterior internodal

Atrioventricular (AV) node

Middle internodal

Posterior internodal

Right atrium

Right ventricle

Arch of aorta

Bachman's bundle

Left atrium

Atrioventricular (AV) bundle (bundle of His)

Left ventricle

Right and left bundle branches

Purkinje fibers

Anterior view of frontal section

image via opentextbc.ca

Normal Sinus Rhythm

- Each P wave is linked in a 1:1 fashion to each QRS complex (atrial depolarization is always linked to ventricular depolarization).
- The P waves are uniform in shape, indicating that the SA node is the only pacemaker driving atrial depolarization.
- P waves in lead II are normally upright and all the same shape.
- P waves in lead V_1 are normally inverted (or on occasion biphasic) and all the same shape.
- The rhythm is regular (but may vary slightly during respirations)
- The rate ranges between 60 and 100 bpm.

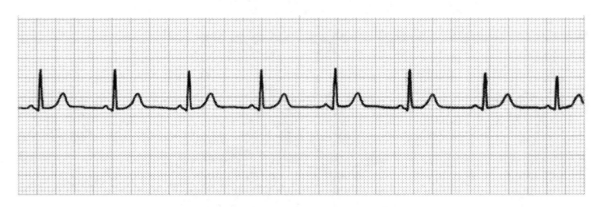

Sinus Brady/AV Blocks

Sinus Bradycardia

- Is identical to normal sinus rhythm, except the rate is less than 60 bpm.
- Cardiac activation starts at the SA node but is slower than normal.
- Sinus bradycardia may be a normal finding in some patients, but in others it is a pathologic finding.

Stable - Asymptomatic (no treatment needed)

- Assess, seek expect consultation
- Obtain patient focused History and Physical

Causes Of Sinus Bradycardia Include:

- Vagal stimulation
- Myocardial infarction
- Hypoxia

- Medications (e.g., β-blockers, calcium channel blockers, digoxin) Metoprolol, verapamil)
- Coronary Artery Disease
- Hypothyroidism
- Iatrogenic illness
- Inflammatory conditions

Signs and Symptoms

Sinus bradycardia may not cause signs or symptoms. However, when sinus bradycardia significantly affects cardiac output, signs and symptoms may include:

- Dizziness or light-headedness
- Syncope
- Fatigue
- Shortness of breath
- Confusion or memory problems

Unstable-Symptomatic (require treatment)

- Assess and maintain airway – provide O_2 as needed
- Vomit- Vital signs, O_2, Monitor, IV assess, Treat
- (Obtain EKG, look for the causes to assist DX and TX.)
- Atropine 1 mg IV Push q 3-5 minutes (max 3 mg)
- May be tried for ALL unstable bradycardias
- Dopamine drip 5-20 mcg/kg/min. Dopamine increases heart rate and contractility
- Epinephrine 2-10 mcg/min (0.1-0.5 mcg/kg/min)
- Prepare for temporary ventricular pacemaker or permanent pacer

APP For Brady's - Atropine, Pacing and/or Pressures

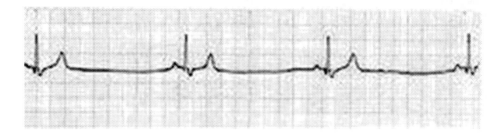

Heart Block

- AV block is partial or complete interruption of impulse transmission from the atria to the ventricles.
- **A**V blocks are classified as first, second or third degree

1st Degree AV Block

- May appear to be a normal sinus rhythm but…. PR interval is > then .20 seconds
- First-degree AV block may be a normal finding in athletes and young patients with high vagal tone.
- It can also be an early sign of degenerative disease of the conduction system or a transient manifestation of myocarditis or drug toxicity.

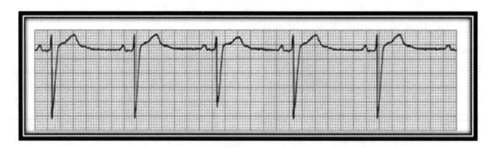

2nd Degree Heart Block (Mobitz Type I (Wenckebach)

- PR interval gets longer and longer until a P wave is not conducted followed by, a dropped QRS.
- In second-degree AV block type I (also called Mobitz type I or Wenckebach block), impulses are delayed and some are not conducted through to the ventricles.
- Conditions or medications that affect the AV node (such as myocarditis, electrolyte abnormalities, inferior wall myocardial infarction or medications such as digoxin) can cause second-degree AV block type I.
- Because the block usually occurs above the bundle of His, conditions or medications that affect the AV node (such as myocarditis, electrolyte abnormalities, inferior wall

myocardial infarction or digoxin) can cause second-degree AV block type I. This type of arrhythmia can also be physiologic.

Signs and Symptoms

- Second-degree AV block type I rarely produces symptoms.
- Some patients may have signs and symptoms of bradycardia.

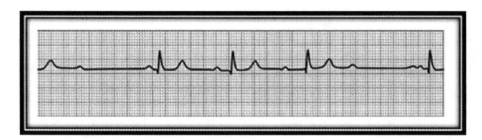

2nd Degree Heart Block (Mobitz Type II)

- PR constant
- More P's than QRS.'s
- As with second-degree AV block type I, some atrial impulses are conducted through to the ventricles, and others are not. However, there are no progressive delays. The blocked impulses may be chaotic or occur in a
- Second-degree AV block type II is always pathologic. It is usually caused by fibrotic disease of the conduction system or anterior wall myocardial infarction.

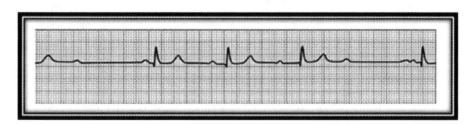

Causes

- Second-degree AV block type II is always pathologic.
- It is usually caused by fibrotic disease of the conduction system or anterior myocardial infarction.

Signs and Symptoms

- Patients may present with light-headedness or syncope, or they may be asymptomatic.
- The clinical presentation varies, depending on the ratio of conducted to blocked impulses.

3rd Degree Heart Block

- No relationship between the PR and QRS, the PR varies
- In third-degree (complete) AV block, no impulses are conducted through to the ventricles.
- Degenerative disease of the conduction system is the leading cause of third-degree AV block. This arrhythmia may also result from damage caused by myocardial infarction, Lyme disease or antiarrhythmic medications.

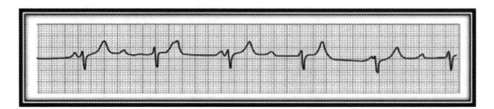

Causes

- Degenerative disease of the conduction system is the leading cause of third-degree AV block.
- This arrhythmia may also result from damage caused by myocardial infarction, Lyme disease or antiarrhythmic drugs.

Signs and Symptoms

- If ventricular contraction is stimulated by pacemaker cells above the bifurcation of the bundle of His, the ventricular rate is relatively fast (40 to 60 bpm) and reliable, and symptoms may be mild (such as fatigue, orthostatic hypotension and effort intolerance).
- If ventricular contraction is stimulated by pacemaker cells in the ventricles, the ventricular rate will be slower (20 to 40 bpm) and less reliable, and symptoms of decreased cardiac output may be more severe (such as syncope).

Common Causes of All AV Block Include

- Fibrosis and scarring of the conduction system and myocardial infarction.
- Medications (such as β-blockers, calcium channel blockers, digoxin and amiodarone)
- Electrolyte abnormalities,
- Myocardial ischemia
- Infectious or inflammatory disorders
- Congenital heart conditions

Blocks Made Simple....Look only at the PR!!!!!

- PR > than .20 = 1 degree AV block
- PR that gets longer, longer, and longer until you have a dropped QRS. = 2nd Degree HB Type I
- PR is constant, never changes = 2nd degree HB type II
- PR all over the place, no consistency = 3rd Heart Block /complete heart Block

Transcutaneous Pacing

- Temporary cardiac pacing using pads or paddles applied externally to the chest

Uses/Indications

- Bradycardia unresponsive to drug therapy
- 3rd degree heart block
- Mobitz type II second-degree heart block when hemodynamically unstable or operation planned
- Overdrive pacing

Method of Insertion And /Or Use

- Place pads in AP position (black on anterior chest, red on posterior chest
- Connect ECG leads
- Set pacemaker to demand
- Turn pacing rate to > 30 bpm above patients intrinsic rhythm
- Set mA to 70
- Start pacing and increase mA until pacing rate captured on monitor
- If pacing rate not captured at a current of 120-130 mA > relocate electrodes and repeat the above.
- Once pacing captured, set current at 5-10 mA above threshold

Complications

- Failure to pace and failure to capture
- Discomfort (pacing is painful)

Sample Strips

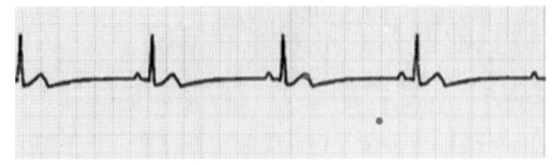

Sinus Brady

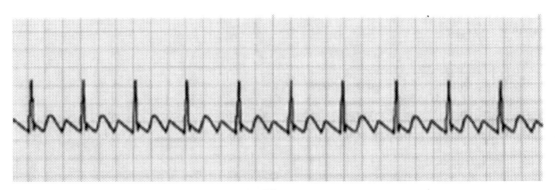

A Flutter

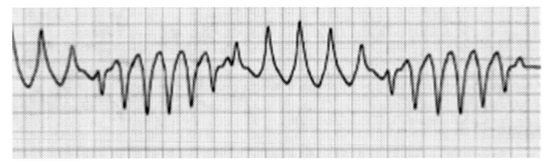

Torades

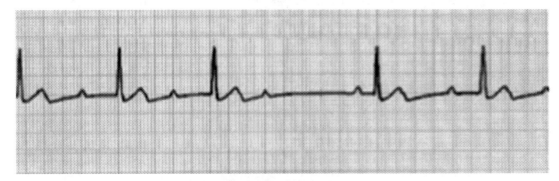

Wenckebach's Block

Tachycardia –Narrow or Wide???

Narrow-Complex (Supraventricular)

- Tachyarrhythmia include sinus tachycardia, atrial flutter and atrial fibrillation.

Wide-Complex Tachyarrhythmia's

- Originate in the ventricles and include ventricular tachycardia (monomorphic and polymorphic), torades de pointes (a form of polymorphic ventricular tachycardia) and ventricular fibrillation.
- The cardiac arrest rhythms—pulseless ventricular tachycardia and ventricular fibrillation—Supraventricular tachycardia with aberrant conduction can also produce a wide-complex tachyarrhythmia.

Sinus Tachycardia is the most common tachyarrhythmia.

- On ECG, sinus tachycardia appears the same as sinus rhythm, except the heart rate is between 100 and 150 bpm.
- Rhythm: regular (atrial and ventricular)
- Rate: 100 to 150 bpm (atrial and ventricular)
- P wave: precedes every QRS. complex
- QRS. complex: < 0.12 second, regular
- T wave: normal
- PR interval: 0.12 to 0.20 second
- QT interval: < 0.46 second

Treat the Cause Underlying Cause First, It Is Most Likely a Systemic One

- Hypovolemia
- Anxiety
- Cold /cough /Fever
- Respiratory distress
- First sign of Shock

Sinus Tachycardia

- Is a normal physiologic response when the body is under stress (such as that caused by exercise, illness or pain).
- When it is a pathophysiologic response, it may be associated with heart failure, lung disease, shock or hyperthyroidism.

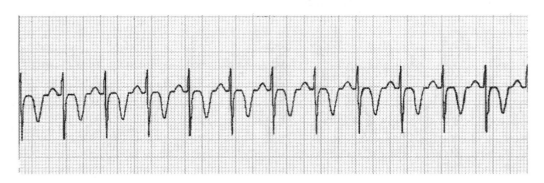

Tachycardia With Pulse Are Either Stable Or Unstable?

Stable

- Assess and maintain airway – provide O2 if hypoxemic
- Vomit- Vital signs, O2, Monitor, IV assess, Treat
- Obtain EKG, look for the causes to assist DX and TX.
- Is rhythm regular or irregular?
- Is QRS wide or narrow?

Unstable... All Unstable Tachycardia Require Synchronized Cardioversion

- Hypotension (systolic B/P < 90)
- Altered LOC
- Chest pain,
- Acute heart failure
- S/S shock

Stable Tachycardia (Narrow QRS) (SVT, A Fib, A-Flutter)

- EKG/Expert consultation
- Vagal Maneuvers

- For SVT

- Adenosine 6 mg (IV slam, followed with a flush with 20 ml NS rapid slam)
- May repeat with Adenosine 12 mg in 1-2 minute
- Anticipate Side effects
- Adenosine slows conduction through the AV node
- Identify underlying rhythm

SVT A general term for tachyarrhythmia that originate above the ventricles in the atria or atrioventricular node and run normally through the bundle branches, producing a normal QRS complex

Atrial Fib/Flutter Narrow Irregular Atrial Fibrillation

- The two key features of atrial fibrillation on ECG are the absence of discrete P waves and the presence of irregularly irregular QRS complexes. The baseline appears flat or undulates slightly, producing, fib waves.
- Rhythm: irregularly irregular (atrial and ventricular)
- Rate: >350 bpm (atrial), 40 to 250 bpm (ventricular)
- P wave: not identifiable (fibrillation waves)
- QRS complex: irregularly irregular
- T wave: not identifiable
- PR interval: unmeasurable
- QT interval: unmeasurable

Atrial Fibrillation is caused by multiple ectopic foci in the atria that cause the atria to contract at a rate of 350 to 600 bpm. Rarely, the atrial rate may be as high as 700 bpm.

- A fib is the absence of discrete P waves and presence of irregularly irregular QRS complexes
- The AV node only allows some of the impulses to pass through to the ventricles, generating an irregularly irregular rhythm that is completely chaotic and unpredictable
- Atrial fibrillation can occur in young patients with no history of cardiac disease.
- Acute alcohol toxicity can precipitate an episode of atrial fibrillation in otherwise healthy patients ("holiday heart syndrome").
- However, atrial fibrillation commonly occurs in the presence of underlying heart disease, lung disease, hyperthyroidism or myocardial infarction.
- Patients with atrial fibrillation may be asymptomatic. However, ventricular rates greater than 100 bpm are usually not tolerated well because the filling time for the ventricles is significantly reduced.
- Symptoms may include shortness of breath, palpitations, chest pain, light-headedness, dizziness and fatigue. In extreme cases, hypotension, syncope and heart failure can occur
  - Goal is, rate control
  - Ca blockers, Verapamil, Cardizem, Beta Blocker, Digoxin

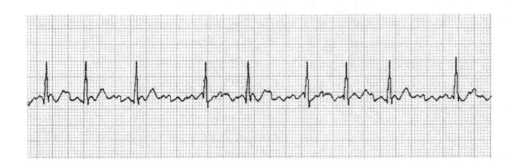

Atrial Flutter is caused by an ectopic focus in the atria that causes the atria to contract at a rate of 250 to 350 bpm. The underlying mechanism of atrial flutter is most often a re-entrant circuit that encircles the tricuspid valve annulus.

- In atrial flutter, atrial contraction occurs at such a rapid rate that discrete P waves separated by a flat baseline cannot be seen. Instead, the baseline continually rises and falls, producing the "flutter" waves.
- In leads II and III, the flutter waves may be quite prominent, creating a "saw tooth" pattern. Because of the volume of atrial impulses, the AV node allows only some of the impulses to pass through to the ventricles.
- In atrial flutter, a 2:1 ratio is the most common (i.e., for every two flutter waves, only one impulse passes through the AV node to generate a QRS complex).
- Ratios of 3:1 and 4:1 are also frequently seen.
- Rhythm: regular (atrial); usually regular but may be irregular (ventricular)
- Rate: 250 to 350 bpm (atrial), 60 to 100 bpm (ventricular; dependent on degree of AV block)
- P wave: sawtooth pattern
- QRS complex: < 0.12 second, regular
- T wave: not identifiable
- PR interval: unmeasurable
- QT interval: unmeasurable
- This rhythm is often seen in patients with heart disease (such as heart failure, rheumatic heart disease or coronary artery disease) or as a postoperative complication.
- Patients may be asymptomatic or present with shortness of breath, palpitations, effort intolerance, chest constriction, weakness or syncope.

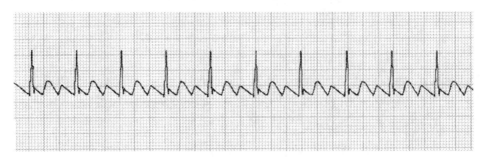

Ventricular Tachycardia occurs when a ventricular focus below the bundle of His becomes the new pacemaker.

- The ventricles contract rapidly (usually at a rate faster than 100 bpm) and usually with a regular rhythm.
- The rapid ventricular rate significantly diminishes cardiac output and can only be sustained for a short period before the patient becomes hemodynamically compromised.
- Ventricular tachycardia can quickly turn into ventricular fibrillation, leading to cardiac arrest.
- Ventricular tachycardia usually occurs in the presence of heart disease or damage, such as that caused by acute or remote myocardial infarction or cardiomyopathy.
- There is a significant risk for ventricular tachycardia after myocardial infarction, and this risk can last for weeks, months or years.
- Ventricular tachycardia may also be precipitated by medications that prolong the QT interval, including amiodarone or other antiarrhythmic and certain antibiotics and antidepressants.
- Electrolyte derangements (including hypocalcemia, hypomagnesemia and hypokalemia) can also be involved.

Stable Tachycardia

Monomorphic V - Tach with a Pulse Wide Regular QRS. Tachy

- In ventricular tachycardia, the QRS. complexes are wide (lasting longer than 120 milliseconds) and bizarre in shape.
- When there is only one ectopic focus in the ventricles, monomorphic ventricular tachycardia is seen on the ECG (i.e., the QRS. complexes are generally the same bizarre shape).
- Rhythm: indiscernible (atrial), usually regular (ventricular)
- Rate: unmeasurable (atrial), > 100 bpm (ventricular)
- P wave: usually absent
- QRS. complex: > 0.12 second, bizarre
- T wave: opposite direction from QRS. complex
- PR interval: unmeasurable
- QT interval: unmeasurable

Treatment

- Consider an antiarrhythmic infusion and expert consultation
- Amiodarone bolus (150 mg in D5W over 10 mins)
- Amiodarone drip 1mg/min for 6 hours then decrease to 0.5 mg/min x 18 hrs.

- Procainamide 20-50 mg/min until arrhythmia suppresses max dose or side effects May follow with drip 1-4 mg/min
- Procainamide delays repolarization and slightly increases the QT interval
- Procainamide when used to treat a stable VT can cause torades
- Sotalol 100 mg(1.5 mg/kg) over 5 minutes

Adenosine may be used for a stable regular monomorphic tachycardia to slow and identify the underlying rhythm

Polymorphic VT - Wide Irregular Tachy

- In polymorphic ventricular tachycardia, which occurs when there are two or more ectopic foci, the QRS. complexes vary in shape and rate.
- Torsades de pointes, a type of polymorphic ventricular tachycardia, has a readily identifiable "party streamer" shape. The QRS. complexes appear to pivot around the isoelectric line, deflecting upward and then downward, with their amplitude becoming smaller and larger, then smaller again.
- The rate is faster than 200 bpm and the rhythm may be regular or irregular.
- P waves are not visible, and the QRS. complexes are wide (lasting longer than 120 milliseconds) and difficult to measure.
- Rhythm: indiscernible (atrial), irregular (ventricular)
- Rate: unmeasurable (atrial), > 100 bpm (ventricular)
- P wave: absent
- QRS. complex: > 0.12 second, bizarre
- T wave: abnormal morphology

Treatment

- Magnesium 1-2 Gm in 50-100 ml D_5W over 5-20 minutes
- If becomes unstable de-fibrillate with 120-200 J
- Hypocalcemia, hypomagnesemia are common causes of V-tach

Unstable Tachycardia

- With sustained ventricular tachycardia, signs and symptoms of reduced cardiac output and hemodynamic compromise develop, including chest pain, hypotension and loss of consciousness

SVT, A Fib, A-Flutter, V Tach with a pulse

Synchronized Cardioversion (all unstable tachycardia's)

- SVT 50-100 J
- A-flutter 50-100 J
- V-tach with a pulse 100 J
- A-Fib 120-200 J

Supraventricular Tachycardia with Aberrant Conduction

- A wide-complex tachyarrhythmia is most often ventricular tachycardia. However, a supraventricular tachycardia with aberrant conduction can also produce wide QRS complexes on ECG.

To Make the Distinction and Definitively Diagnose Ventricular Tachycardia,

- 12-lead ECG is needed.
- Lead V_1 on a 5-lead ECG can also be helpful to differentiate a wide-complex ventricular tachycardia from supraventricular tachycardia with aberrant conduction.
- AV dissociation is pathognomonic for supraventricular tachycardia with aberrant conduction.
- The following are validated criteria for proving ventricular tachycardia with a high degree of specificity (greater than 90%).
- If any one of these criteria is met, treat the arrhythmia as stable ventricular tachycardia.
- Note that although these criteria can assist with diagnosing ventricular tachycardia, they are of little use in ruling it out.
- In other words, even if none of these criteria are met, the patient may still have ventricular tachycardia. Before treating suspected ventricular tachycardia with medications, you must be confident that the rhythm is ventricular tachycardia. If in doubt and the patient's condition permits, seek expert consultation

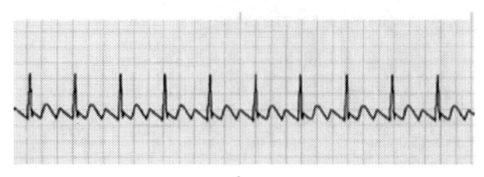

A Flutter

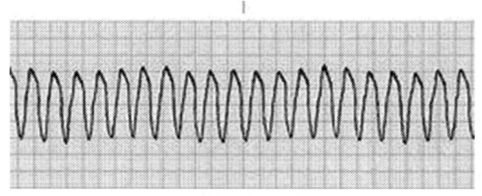

V Tach with a Pulse

Defibrillation (Only For Pts with NO Pulse)

Pulseless V-Tach/Fib/Torades

- 120 j - 200 j

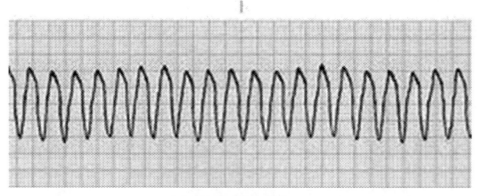

V- Tach No Pulse

Cardiac Arrest

Shock vs No Shock

- Dead…Top Priority High Quality CPR

Shockable (Alt shock/med)

VF, Pulseless V Tach, Torsade's

- Early de-fib (120-200 J) then no matter whatever is going on shock q2 minutes
- Continue compressions while charging (it produces a small amt. of blood flow to help the shock to be more effective)
- Safe de-fib-remove blow by O2, verbalize all clear, eyes on patient
- Ok to use AED in Snow…if in water remove pt., dry off then shock
- Back on chest immediately after shocking (30:2)
- reassess rhythm in 2 minutes pulse check only if rhythm changes
- Obtain IV/IO access – the first drug that dead adults and only dead adults get is Epinephrine 1 mg IVP Q 3-5 minutes (drugs are giving during compressions/try to give at the beginning of the cycle to allow for circulation)
- Second drug-antiarrhythmic Amiodarone 300 mg (give between the 1st and 2nd epi dose) can repeat with 150 mg in 3-5 minutes
- Lidocaine an antiarrhythmic can be used instead of Amiodarone. Dose 1-1.5 mg /kg IVP…May repeat in 10-15 minutes with ½ of the initial dose .Infusion dose 1-4 mg/min start at 1 mg higher that the total bolus given
- Lidocaine can be use in people with or without a pulse Max dose 3 mg/kg
- Suspect hyperkalemia in all patients with acute or chronic renal failure who exhibit a wide-complex ventricular rhythm or tall, peaked T waves on an ECG before cardiac arrest.
- Precipitating causes of ventricular fibrillation include electrocution, myocardial ischemia or infarction, shock, stimulant overdose and ventricular tachycardia

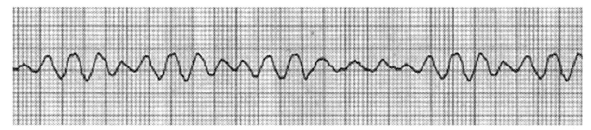

V Fib

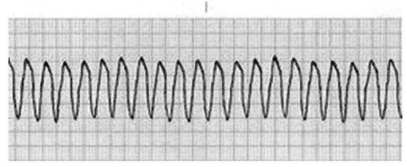

V Tach

Cardiac Arrest

Cardiac Arrest No Shock (Dead)

- Top Priority High Quality CPR
- PEA or Asystole

PEA - organize rhythm on the monitor (may even look like a normal sinus but…no detectable pulse

Asystole – confirm in 2 leads!!!

- Treatment is the same for both
  - High quality CPR
  - Epi mg Q 3-5 minutes
  - Between Epi doses search for H & T's
  - For known acidosis consider Na Bicarb

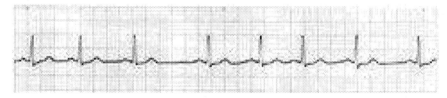

Regular Rhythm No Pulse /PEA

Administering Medications during a Cardiac Arrest

- All medications administrated through the IV or intraosseous infusion route should be followed by a 10- to 20-mL fluid bolus.
- Intraosseous (IO) access is often used as an alternative to IV access in emergency situations
- As with IV access, IO access can be used to administer medications, fluids and blood products and to collect blood for laboratory analysis

- Medication dosing is the same for IO and IV
- Since 2015, no new studies were identified, so the 2015 recommendation of standard dose epinephrine remains unchanged.
- 2019 Recommendation: It is recommended that epinephrine be administered for cardiac arrest
- The benefits of epinephrine support the recommendation for its use, despite some remaining uncertainty about overall impact on neurological outcome.
- Vasopressin may be considered in cardiac arrest, but it offers no advantage as a substitute for epinephrine.
- Vasopressin combined with epinephrine may be considered in cardiac arrest, but it offers no advantage as a substitute for epinephrine alone.

Post Cardiac Arrest ROSC

- Optimization of brain function is the primary goal of post–cardiac arrest care. Ensuring adequate mean arterial pressure and controlling intracranial pressure optimize cerebral perfusion

Post-Cardiac Arrest, Focuses on Support Of:

- Neurologic function, including Targeted Temperature Management
- Circulation, including treatment of possible acute coronary occlusion (ie, ST-elevation myocardial infarction), arrhythmias and shock, and support of fluid balance

Conduct A Primary Assessment And Perform Initial Interventions, Including:

- Establishing cardiac monitoring
- Pulse oximetry
- Capnography
- Noninvasive blood pressure monitoring or arterial pressure monitoring
- 12-lead ECG
- Obtaining blood samples for laboratory testing

Airway

- Ensure oxygenation and ventilation
- Consider an advance airway/verify tube placement
- Waveform capnography (35-40 during ROSC)
- In ROSC, Maint O2 sat 92-98% (prolong use of high FIO2 can cause oxygen toxicity)
- Do not hyperventilate- hyperventilation decreases CO/ cerebral perfusion

- ABG's Chest x-ray

Breathing / Rescue breathing

- 1 breath q 6 seconds/10 BPM…Adults
- 1 breath q 2-3 second/20-30 BPM….Children and infants

Circulation

- Optimize cardiac output, stroke volume (preload, contractility and afterload)
- Monitor and treat SBP < 90 give fluids NS or LR 1-2 L …
- Monitor heart rate, treat arrhythmias
- Dopamine 2-20 mcg/kg/min or Epi (0.1-0.5 mcg/kg/min) IV/IO
- Poor myocardial function inotropes

D- Neuro Deceit

- Assess for secondary brain injury related to hypoxia/ hypotension/ hypoglycemia
- Follow commands if not consider TTM 34-36 degrees celuis for at least 24 hours a various of methods can be used including administering an ice-cold IV fluid bolus (30 mL/kg), using endovascular catheters or employing surface cooling strategies (e.g., cooling blankets, ice packs).

E- EKG ASAP (R/O Stemi),

- TX to a facility that does PCI
- Labs DX test
- Look for treatable causes

Top priority after ROSC – is Oxygenation

Clinical Indications of ROSC

- Organized rhythm on the cardiac monitor/defibrillator combined with a palpable central pulse
- Clinical signs of perfusion,
- Sudden increase in the PETCO level,
- PETCO > 40
- Measurable blood pressure and improved skin color
- Patient movement, normal breathing or coughing, arterial pulse waveform on an A-line when no compressions are being delivered

Post–Cardiac Arrest Syndrome (PCAS).

- Is a systemic response to ischemia/reperfusion
- It reflects impaired tissue oxygenation causing systemic inflammation, vascular instability, and increased coagulation along with adrenal Suppression and a lowered resistance to infection.
- Clinical manifestations include: fever, hypotension, hyperglycemia, infection and multi organ failure.

Acute Coronary Syndrome (ACS)

- a general term for a group of life-threatening conditions that occur because of a sudden reduction in blood flow to the heart

Chest Pain Suggestive Of Myocardial Ischemia

- Immediate Assessment (<10 minutes) including 12 lead ECG, VS, O2 Sat, IV Access,
- Rainbow of labs (baseline coagulation studies/electrolytes/cardiac makers/CBC)
- Targeted History and Physical
- Chest x-ray within 30 minutes
- MONA
- 2-4 L/min for O2 Sat's below 90%
- ASA 160-325 mg PO
- Ntg. 0.4 mg SL or spray Vasodilator, decreases preload, watch BP!
- Hold Nitro if hypotensive (SB/P <90) Rt. sided MI or recent erectile enhancement drugs
- Morphine 2-4 MG IV every 5 min for pain not relieved with Ntg. (Use morphine cautiously)
- Treatment of Choice for STEMI: REPERFUSION!!
- Window of Opportunity for STEMI:
- Symptoms Present <12 hrs.
- Angiography with angioplasty or stent placement

Primary Percutaneous Coronary Intervention (PCI)

- Performed as the first line therapy for ST-segment elevation myocardial infarction (STEMI)
- Transport to PCI capable facility
- GOAL – Time of first medical contact, to PCI reperfusion <90 min.

Thrombolytic Therapy

- If not a candidate for Cardiac Catheterization
- GOAL– Door to Thrombolytic Drug < 30 min
- An early invasive strategy should be considered for patients with high-risk non–ST-segment elevation acute coronary syndromes (NSTE-ACS). Elevated serum cardiac markers
- ST segment. Represents the time between the end of ventricular depolarization and the beginning of ventricular repolarization. It is measured from the end of the QRS complex to the beginning of the T wave

Stroke

- Is the fifth-leading cause of death and is a leading cause of long-term disability.
- Each year approximately about one stroke occurs every 40 seconds.
- Among people experiencing a stroke, one third will die, one third will have long term disability and one third will recover with minimal or no disability.

Early Management of Acute Stroke Is Included In ACLS Training

- Just as with cardiac emergencies, time is a critical component of treatment.
- Timely recognition, assessment and management of acute stroke can minimize brain injury and improve patient outcomes.
- Stroke is a sudden neurologic deficit that occurs because of impaired blood flow to part of the brain.

Stroke Has Four Defining Features:

- A sudden onset of signs and symptom
- Primary involvement of the central nervous system
- Lasting neurologic deficit
- A vascular cause

Two Main Types of Stroke: Ischemic and Hemorrhagic.

Ischemic Stroke

- Occurs when a blood vessel supplying the brain is occluded
- An embolic stroke occurs when a plaque fragment or blood clot forms elsewhere within the circulatory system and travels to the cerebral circulation. Often the source of the embolus is a blood clot that forms in the heart or the large arteries in the upper

chest or neck. Between 15% and 20% of embolic strokes are associated with atrial fibrillation.

- For acute ischemic stroke, the goal of treatment is to relieve the obstruction and restore blood flow to the brain tissue.
- Acute ischemic stroke can be treated with fibrinolytic therapy, endovascular therapy or both, but the window for treatment is narrow.
- 87% of strokes are ischemic

Hemorrhagic Stroke

- Occurs when a weakened blood vessel in the brain ruptures and pressure from the bleeding damages the brain tissue. This type of stroke is frequently caused by hypertension or aneurysms.
- Hemorrhagic strokes can be classified as intracerebral or subarachnoid.

Subarachnoid

- Bleeding onto the surface of the brain occurs when a blood vessel located on the surface of the brain ruptures, causing bleeding into the subarachnoid space.
- This type of hemorrhage is most often caused by a ruptured aneurysm but can also be caused by an arteriovenous malformation, bleeding disorder, head injury or anticoagulant therapy.

Intracerebral

- Bleeding in the brain intracerebral hemorrhage, the most common form of hemorrhagic stroke, occurs when an artery located within the brain bursts, causing bleeding into the surrounding brain tissue.
- Intracerebral hemorrhage may be caused by an arteriovenous malformation.
- Can be fatal at onset, hypertension most common precipitating factor

8 D's of Stroke

Detection:

- Early recognize signs and symptoms

Dispatch:

- Early activation of EMS

Delivery:

- Pre-hospital EMS assessment done using the Cincinnati Pre-Hospital Stroke Score
- Glucose pre hospital and rechecked upon arrival to the facility
- Identify time symptoms began (alert receiving hospital of the findings)

Door:

- assess within 10 minutes /stroke alert, 3 hr. window of opportunity for thrombolytic
- Select pts may have up to 4.5 hr. window
- Optional treatments may have slightly longer window
- Immediate Assessment - Neurological Screening ASAP, H & P, Glasgow, NIH
- NIH Stoke evaluates level of consciousness, visual function, motor function, sensation and neglect, Cerebellar function and language deficits.
- VS, IV, Complete Blood Count, Electrolytes, Coagulation Studies, Blood Sugar. 12-Lead EKG (R/O Arrhythmia That May Have Caused The Stroke

Data/Decision/Drug /Device:

- CT to R/O bleed: If CT shows NO hemorrhage:
- CT down... Divert to Stroke Center with Head CT capabilities
- CT needs to be done ASAP/25 minute, read within 45 minutes
- Thrombolytic criteria? Clot Retrieval?

Disposition:

- Admission to Stroke Unit or ICU within 3 hrs.
- Endovascular therapy should be initiated within 6 hours

If CT Shows Hemorrhage:

- Consult Neurosurgery, reverse anticoagulation, and/or bleeding disorder, monitor neurological condition, control hypertension Assessment

Clinical Presentation Signs And Symptoms Of Stroke Include:

- Sudden weakness, numbness or tingling on one side of the face or body.
- Sudden onset of confusion.
- Sudden difficulty with language, including difficulty speaking, difficulty understanding or garbled speech
- Sudden vision difficulties in one or both eyes.

- Difficulty with walking, balance or coordination
- Sudden severe headache

Assessment Tools

FAST

- **F-** Facial Droop(have the pt. smile, note if both sides of the face move equally)
- **A-** Arm Drift(have them close their eyes and hold both arms out straight with palms up for 10 seconds)
- **S-** Speech (repeat You can't teach an old dog new tricks)
- **T-** Time Onset of Symptoms

Cincinnati Pre Hospital Stroke Scale (CPSS)

- Used to diagnose a potential stroke in a pre-hospital setting (facial droop, arm drift, abnormal speech)
- One abnormality in the CPSS is associated with a 72% probability of a stroke

Miami Emergency Neurologic Deficit (MEND)

- The MEND checklist assesses three areas (mental status, cranial nerve function and limb function) and provides more detailed information about the severity and location of the stroke.
- It can also be used to establish a baseline of neurologic function for future comparison.
- The MEND checklist may be completed by prehospital providers or hospital providers.

Rapid Arterial Occlusion Evaluation (RACE) Scale

- The RACE scale scores the patient's condition in five areas (facial palsy, arm motor function, leg motor function, head and gaze deviation, and agnosia/aphasia)
- Used by prehospital providers to screen for possible large vessel occlusion.
- A score of 5 or greater indicates possible large vessel occlusion with a sensitivity of 85% and a specificity of 69%.

National Institutes of Health Stroke Scale (NIHSS)

- Can be used to both assess and quantify deficits,
- Should be administered to all patients with suspected stroke once they arrive at the receiving facility.

- The NIHSS evaluates level of consciousness, visual function, motor function, sensation and neglect, cerebellar function and language deficits and helps to determine both the location and the severity of the stroke.
- It can also be used to assess the probability of ischemic stroke.

Blood Glucose

- Is checked out of hospital/and upon arrive to ED
- Hypo/hyperglycemia may alter their neuro status

Time Frames

- Assess within 10 minutes from arrival
- Within 20 minutes, a comprehensive neurologic assessment should be completed and brain imaging should be performed.
- Within 45 minutes the CT should be read.
- "Normal CT start" Fibrinolytic ASAP (Door to drug 45- 60 minutes)
- Fibrinolytic therapy is ideally administered within 3 hours of the onset of symptoms, although this time frame may be extended to 4.5 hours for some patients.
- Endovascular therapy is ideally administered within 6 hours of the onset of symptoms, although this time frame may be extended to 24 hours for some patients

References

- AHA/ARC resuscitation guidelines, 2010, 2015, 2019, 2020
- https://eccguidelines.heart.org
- 2019 American Heart Association Guidelines Update on Adult Advanced Cardiovascular Life Support

Images

- https://opentextbc.ca/anatomyandphysiologyopenstax/chapter/cardiac-muscle-and-electrical-activity/
- Electrical Activity of the Heart: www.cablesandsensors.com
- 3 and 5 EKG lead placement: **Dr Mike Cadogan** - https://litfl.com
- 15 lead EKG Jaakko Malmivuo, Professor www.bem.fi/malmivuo
- 12 lead ECG John Gladstein Medical Device Depot, Inc www.medicaldevicedepot.com

Rhythm strips

- Nancy Smith RN BSN
  AHA Training Center Coordinator, Banner Health Nancy.Smith@bannerhealth.com

Printed in the United States
By Bookmasters